Behind those
care home doors

Behind those
care home doors

How to avoid care 'professionals' with their eyes wide shut

Adeline Dalley

THE CHOIR PRESS

First published in the United Kingdom in 2014 by
The Choir Press

ISBN 978-1-909300-39-2

Contents

Contents

Foreword

I was honoured and delighted when Adeline invited me to write the foreword to her book. I know from personal experience, sadly, how Care and Nursing Homes can fall woefully short of the promises in their glossy brochures and, as a result, my mother, now aged 95, is about to endure her 4th care home move. This is a book that was crying out to be written and, with the recent exposure of abuse of vulnerable people in residential homes, couldn't be more timely. I truly believe that there is nobody better qualified to write it than Adeline. She writes from the heart and with many years as a carer in several care homes she has a solid platform of knowledge and experience. She also writes with the passion of someone who cares deeply about their role in what is often end of life care.

When my mother, Joan Bader, widow of Sir Douglas Bader, suffered a stroke and personal care was no longer viable, we regretfully made the decision to move her into a residential care home.

Sadly the first home didn't suit her (or vice versa!) and we moved her again. It was after this move that I first met Adeline. It was clear from the outset that Adeline is a wonderful carer with a true and, regrettably, all too rare ability to empathise with her elderly residents whatever their needs. She loves her residents like family and this was evident when my mother suffered inadequate care following a second stroke at this care home. Adeline had the courage to safeguard her against a system that is not unknown for closing ranks in these instances and, as a result, my mother was hospitalised and has almost miraculously recovered. We were extremely grateful to Adeline for her courage and writing this foreword is also my way of saying thank you.

I know at first hand the guilt that can accompany the decision to place a loved one in care coupled with the hope that their physical and emotional needs be met as should happen in a good care home whether you are present or not. There is a lot we can do, however, to make sure that the choice of home is right. We can look past the glossy brochures and the promises and talk to those directly involved; the carers and residents themselves. As Adeline says, a lot can be learned about the true nature of the care and staffing levels by asking staff direct questions in the manager's absence. Transparency is certainly a virtue when it comes to care homes and the value of carers being able to talk directly and without fear to residents' families should not be overlooked. Transparency breeds trust and that is vital in this situation. A care home should be what it says – it is intended, after all, to be a home from home but with care and support when that has become necessary.

Hearing how often carers see and even report ill-treatment or neglect in care homes but are ignored or intimidated into silence is frightening, especially as with our ageing population so many people are already in care or will need care in the future. Those with families or friends to look out for and speak for them are the lucky ones but what about those without? Who will be their voice if those looking after them are aware that there is a problem with their care but are afraid to report it? This issue is exacerbated by society's perception of the value of the role of carers and the salaries paid to those performing this difficult and vital task. Frequently they are paid the minimum wage or a figure not far from it even for experienced carers. Care homes are often understaffed as a result and crying out for applicants. How much easier it is then to ignore the situation or walk away into another job than to make a stand, report the problem and then face the consequences. How many will worry more about keeping friends and the status quo, however uncomfortable that may make them, than protecting the residents in their care?

This book hasn't been written by an impersonal professional but an experienced senior carer on the front line, fighting for carers to be listened to so that our vulnerable relatives and loved ones are protected from harm and abuse. Written with passion and considerable background experience, knowledge and wisdom, I would recommend that this book becomes mandatory educational curriculum reading, certainly for the Health and Social Care sector students as well as doctors, nurses and anyone who hopes to make a career involving the care of the elderly. Giving them this insight could potentially make a difference to the care they give and the confidence to recognise and act against poor care standards when they see them and thereby make a difference to people's lives at this critical time.

One thing is certain and that is that we will all die. Many of us will get old and suffer some or all of the afflictions and frailties that go with that first. For me the issue seems to be looming personally at an alarming rate, it's certainly close enough for me to be giving a fair bit of thought to the rest of my life and how I would hope to be able to live it. Yet I can still only begin to imagine how it must feel to be old, frail and dependent. Perhaps to have no sight, or hearing; perhaps to be unable to stand or even sit unaided let alone perform the everyday tasks it's easy to take for granted. To be confused; frightened perhaps by the realisation that you can no longer remember the names or faces of loved ones or other aspects of life previously important to you. To be moved, often against your wishes, from your home to a strange and impersonal care or nursing home. To be facing not just the knowledge that even with the blessing of good health, there are far less years ahead than behind but the approach of death itself. To me the prospect is terrifying and, as Adeline says in her book, good end of life care is vitally important and is the last gift we can give to somebody whatever their situation. We should strive to ensure that that care is available to all. We are looked after when we are babies, equally we should be secure in the knowledge that we'll be looked after when we become frail and dependent at the other end of our lives with our dignity respected and preserved.

As this book needed to be written, it also needs to be read by all, young and old. Care tutors and lecturers, care managers and companies, care students, healthcare professionals, people looking at care homes as well as governing bodies who monitor care homes. As good care starts at the top, managers in particular should take note.

Sir Douglas, my stepfather, believed passionately in fairness and went out of his way to help and encourage vulnerable people. I have no doubt that he would be horrified at the treatment meted out to some of the most vulnerable in our society and that he would have approved wholeheartedly of Adeline's effort to make this a thing of the past by writing this book. Thank you for putting into words what so many of us think, Adeline.

Wendy McCleave

Preface

One of the hardest decisions we may have to make in our lives is the decision that our loved one needs professional care.

The tail end of our lives is as important as the beginning, when we were unable to communicate and relied on loving people to identify and provide for our every need. That love and patience is needed again now, and families are relying on the care home they choose to meet these needs. So why are so many places failing this task? My experiences in too many care settings are frightening proof of this failure, and it needs to stop. Care needs to change for the better, and fast.

The idea of this book is to advise people on what to look for in a good care home, and what to expect. There are, I am sure, many care homes that are as wonderful as the one I am in now; however, there are some that are really to be avoided. My aim is not to scare people choosing care, but to educate them, as someone who knows the profession, on seeing beyond what so many people see as a good environment.

Although there are many good books by doctors and nurses, it is the carers who in my experience spend the most time with the residents, caring for their needs. Despite this, we are often ignored because some staff class us as 'just a carer'. With poor care standards having been highlighted recently in the press, I hope my experiences in care will help others to realise how we need to change the way care is provided.

This book is aimed at anyone in a care setting already, including managers and care groups. It is also for individuals looking to place a family member into care, or anyone thinking of starting a care career.

In this book I share some very negative experiences which could have led me to cease working in the care industry, had I not found my current position.

Relatives' guilt trip

One of the most common things a loved one in need of care might say to us is, 'Don't ever put me in a care home.'

When you hear this, the questions going through your mind feel endless. That little guilt trip is probably setting in; you know, the one that says 'should you be taking on a full carer's role for your loved one?'

In reality many people will not be able to accomplish this. There are jobs, children, grandchildren and financial restrictions to consider. Sadly many more people are now suffering with dementia and other memory-restricting illnesses requiring specialised care.

Although it may seem selfish, there is also your own health to consider. I have met many families at breaking point because they have been trying to juggle family life and care of a loved one. This can

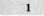

result in a breakdown from exhaustion, which will affect your ability to cope.

At 15 I was volunteering with the Red Cross, helping the elderly with shopping and housework. As soon as school was finished I went into care, and after 16 years I have never looked back. When having my children I did part-time care work and studied care courses, and now I am working full-time in palliative care while my husband looks after our children; he understands how committed I am in my career choice and in my passion to strive for good care.

Having had so many let-downs from care managers and nurses in my past, my aim is to show the importance of good care. More people are living longer than ever before and there is such a huge need for carers and nurses. There are two things I am hoping I will be able to convey through my book as someone who has experienced many homes. Firstly, this book will hopefully help loved ones facing the care dilemma and give them an idea of what to expect; secondly, I want all current carers as well as those considering going into care to realise what is needed to make a care home successful and how to improve their standards.

Another area I feel the Care Quality Commission (CQC) need to look at is safe staffing levels, especially when carrying out an inspection. This is crucial to getting a true picture of the care setting and improving care standards.

Abuse in care – recognition and action

This may be your main concern when placing a loved one into care. Abuse comes under many categories, but this book offers a basic and easy-to-understand guide for staff as well as relatives on spotting the signs and how to act.

All types of abuse can be carried out by anyone: management, carers, social workers, relatives and friends, neighbours, priests, anyone who has contact with the victim. Also important, though, are the cases where people are confused and mistakenly say abuse has happened; we will talk about this a bit more in a minute.

There are people who may feel brave enough to tell us if they are suffering abuse; however, we must always be aware of signs from people who don't feel they can speak out.

The hardest situation as a member of care home staff is when someone tells you they have been abused but begs you not to say anything for fear of reprisals. It would be wrong to agree to this because it is our duty of care to protect our residents and report a disclosure. The best thing to do if you are told about abuse is to document everything you can, so it can be passed on to help an investigation.

Who should you go to? This will depend on who the accused is; if a manager of the care home has been accused of abuse then you may go to the regional director. If you feel nobody in the home will act or if various people have been accused then a couple of your options are to contact your Local Authority Safeguarding Team or CQC for advice.

For all care workers there should be advice in your contract on concerns and whistle-blowing policies.

Types of abuse and possible signs

Everyone needs to remember that the person being abused needs protecting and this is our main priority.

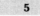

There are many people who, upon realising that they are working in a care setting where abuse is happening, will just leave for a new job or rely on the hope that someone else will speak out. Ignoring the situation like this makes them nearly as bad as the abuser, in my opinion. It would be a similar situation if as a relative you were to take your loved one out of a home where you knew abuse was happening and said nothing to anyone; just stop and think of all the people left behind. If it were your mum or dad you would want someone to protect them, wouldn't you?

Types of abuse include:

- *Physical abuse:* when someone hurts you physically in the flesh, for example by hitting or pinching you, forcing you to take medication when you don't want to. Bruising, cuts and burns may be visible, but not always. When a resident has no explanation for their injuries this may be a concern.

- *Financial abuse:* when someone takes or uses your belongings or money without asking you. Money may go missing, payments may be made for other people's things and the victim may not be able to say how their money has been spent.

If valuables go missing, there are unexplained money worries, the resident has less money than they are used to and maybe mysterious payments appear on bank statements, these could be signs of this type of abuse.

- *Sexual abuse:* this is when someone is forced to take part in sexual activities/acts against their wishes, being touched or being forced to touch someone else in a sexual way. Changes in behaviour, physical discomfort, fear of getting personal hygiene needs tended to, genital infections etc. may be signs of this.

- *Psychological abuse:* when people say unkind things and hurt your feelings, or threaten you in any way. Calling names, controlling your choices, ignoring your requests and blaming you for things. Confusion, fear, anxiety and disturbed sleep can be signs of this type of abuse.

- *Discriminatory abuse:* suffering abuse because you are a particular race, religion etc. or are just different to others. You may be gay or lesbian or may not speak English as a first language, for instance. If the needs of certain residents are not met, correct foods are not provided etc., this may be a sign of discriminatory abuse in the care home; there could also be signs of isolation, withdrawal, anxiety from not having choices upheld.

* *General neglect:* when care and support needs are not met. There may be unclean bedding on the bed and dirty clothes on the resident. Residents may be unwashed, hungry or thirsty and too cold. Deterioration in the appearance and health of the patient are possible signs.

* *Institutional abuse:* this is when there is frequently or consistently poor care in hospitals and care settings. People have to go to bed and get up when it suits staff; people have no choice on wash times; there may be a lack of activities, and requests to speak to family are not met. Often you can tell if there are not enough staff on. Routines and procedures are favoured over the person, and call bells may be left ringing for a long time. This often is shown by residents becoming withdrawn and depressed, experiencing low feelings and thoughts.

Any good care home would rather look into an accusation of abuse that turns out to be unfounded than miss true abuse of a patient. Years ago a patient told me and two other staff members that people had been in her room touching each other and involving her; the two other staff members and I all gave full details of this to the nurse in charge. Next the same patient accused a nurse of giving her the wrong medication. The people accused in the first instance had not been on duty when the assault was said to have taken place and the nurse accused of giving incorrect medication was on holiday that week. The fact that this patient was hallucinating and had a high temperature as well made us suspicious of an infection. The GP was in for the round that day and the lady had a nasty urine infection; after antibiotics she was back to her normal happy self again. So when you are visiting your relative and feel there is a change that concerns you in any way, speak to staff in charge, who should be more than happy to investigate in any way necessary.

Choosing the right home – what to ask

If you are looking for a home for your loved one, beware of the brochure with the wonderful pictures and loving words of comfort. Hardly ever have I been able to see a brochure being true to its fancy promises of the care your loved one will receive.

You should also think carefully about what the manager is telling you and how close to the truth this could be. I have many times felt a failure when managers have walked past me with potential clients, giving the usual spiel on what good quality of care/food their loved one will receive. I have stood there helplessly, knowing how untruthful these facts are and wanting to tell it how it is. In one of the worst ever homes I worked in, when staff had to do the tours, I actually said to some visitors to look elsewhere as the home was awful; they asked me whether I would put my nan in the home and no, I will not lie. I have watched too many twists of the truth. Anyone would want to know if it were their loved one going into a home, and I am sure they would have respect for anyone telling the truth about the home. Don't be afraid to ask staff questions rather than management; a good manager who has been honest will have no problem with this.

Unfortunately, it can be difficult to find out whether concerns have previously been raised regarding the care in a particular home. Should anyone contact a local authority safeguarding team with concerns about a patient's care, an investigation should be carried out as this is a safeguarding alert and their duty is to protect the vulnerable. What I find worrying is the fact that if the CQC become involved with looking at compliances in a care home after an alert, they do not have to visit the care home themselves; apparently the verdict is down to the inspector's judgement. Not only that, but safeguarding concerns raised will not appear on any report on the CQC website; only compliance issues that were failed will be published, even if a few different alerts have been received regarding a particular care setting. I have been advised that anyone could contact their local authority, but there is no guarantee that they will deliver information that they hold on concerns raised regarding a particular home. I don't believe that personal information should be published, but surely, if we are looking for a home for our parents to live in, we have the right to see if anyone has raised concerns. What I have found in so many previous homes is that there are staff striving, wanting to care, but staff higher up the chain have their eyes wide shut to the idea of giving real care, cutting corners with no thought for those suffering these consequences.

I decided after all these years that I will not work anywhere I am not happy with the care given, or with the truthfulness of the care company on its standards when advertising to potential clients. A good company will appreciate honesty from staff, patients and patients' relatives, as this shows true passion for good care.

Here are some points to consider that should help you choose the right home for your loved one:

Location

- Are family and friends able to get there easily?

- Are there any local shops your relative can visit nearby?

- Are there any noisy pubs within earshot? Is it on a busy road?

- Does the home have a garden for residents to sit/help in?

- Is the home and garden accessible for wheel-chairs via ramps, lifts etc.?

- Does the garden look well kept?

Safety and security

- Do they have fire procedures, plans of action?

- Is the garden secure to stop strangers coming in or residents wandering?

- Are window opening restrictions in place to prevent falls?

- What are the secure access procedures in place for residents' safety and visitors to get in and out?

- Are there hand rails in place around the home for residents?

- Is there air conditioning for comfort in hot weather?

Living space

- Can residents choose their own room?

- Can prospective residents stay for a week to see if they like it?

- Can they bring their own furniture and pictures?

- Do the rooms look bright and clean with space to walk around safely?

- Can residents choose when they wish to stay in their rooms?

- Are there pets in the home? Can pets be brought in for visits?

- Do staff members knock on doors before entering?

- Is there a room where relatives can make drinks for themselves and their loved one?

- Does the bedroom have good storage space?

- Is the en suite clean and accessible?

- Are staff trained and tactful when dealing with incontinence episodes, assisting people to the toilet, bathing, showering?

Lounges and communal areas

- Are chairs clean and comfy, arranged in small groups to encourage chatting?

- Is there a quieter lounge where people can go with relatives for quieter time or if they have had enough of TV?

- Are there accessible toilets near the communal areas that are clearly visible?

- Do these areas have a call bell system for assistance?

Dining areas

- Are special diets and likes and dislikes catered for?

- How many choices are there at meal times?

- If someone is hungry can they eat, day or night?

- Do the tables, cloths and cutlery look clean and tidy?

- Can you see the current menu?

- Do staff sensitively assist people who need encouragement with eating or actually need to be fed?

- Can meals be taken in your room if wanted?

Visitors

- Can you visit at any time?

- If your loved one is poorly can you stay with them overnight?

- Can family join in outings/activities?

- Can children visit?

- If booked, can you have a meal with a loved one?

- Is there a relatives' meeting where everyone gets together to talk about the home and its care with the manager?

- Can the manager be contacted at any time if there is a serious concern?

Activities

- Are there activities formulated specially for dementia patients?

- Can residents choose which activities they want to participate in?

- Is there a changing weekly schedule of activities?

- Can residents listen to music if they wish?

- How are special occasions like birthdays celebrated?

- Can residents help staff with jobs like tidying linen cupboards to feel useful and needed?

Health changes and your involvement

- Will you be contacted if your relative is poorly/has a fall?

- Can you choose your own GP?

- How often are medical notes and medications reviewed? If there are changes, will you be contacted?

- Does the home have access to hairdressers, chiropodists, beauticians, eyesight screening and audiology? If appointments are outside the home, will they arrange transport and send staff as an escort?

General impressions

- On arrival, was everyone friendly and polite?

- Does the home feel welcoming? Your own instincts matter too.

- Does the home have a pleasant smell, no nasty odours?

- Does it look clean, fresh and well maintained?

- At any point did you feel under pressure to say whether you would definitely choose that home? Any good care setting will welcome questions and be happy for you to go away and think. A good home will also realise how important this decision is for you and the future of your relative.

Residents you see around the home

- Do not be afraid to speak if residents say hello and try to converse; ask them how they like the home.

- Do you see staff speaking kindly to the residents?

- Are the residents clean and well dressed?

- Do they look alert and interested in their surroundings?

- While you are there, are the residents doing anything? This may be time-dependent.

- Listen; are there call bells going off? Does this go on for long?

- Have you seen staff encouraging people to do what they can? Taking the easy option by putting people who can still walk in a wheelchair may de-skill people and cause them to lose the movement/independence they have left.

- Do residents have access to drink nearby if they want it?

- Is the call bell within the reach of the residents?

Staff

- Do staff have experience and regular training?

- Is there an appropriate skills mix on shifts?

- Are staff encouraged to sit and chat with residents?

- Have staff members that have seen you acknowledged you?

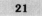

- What is done to ensure staff learn about residents' backgrounds, habits and interests?

- Will your relative have a key worker?

- Is there always someone available to discuss any concerns with?

Managers and deputies

- Does the manager have a friendly manner towards residents and staff? (Care staff are as good as management because they are the people controlling care standards and working conditions.)

- Are they open when asked questions? Do they take your questions seriously?

- Do they have a good knowledge of the type of care the home may specialise in?

Contracts

If the local authorities are involved with funding they may have a contract with the home and you should ask to see a copy. If you are independently arranging a home for your loved one then it may be worth speaking to the Citizen's Advice Bureau or a solicitor first for advice on contracts. Some things to be sure on:

- In the weekly fee what is included, what notice is given if fees are raised and what may be charged as extras?

- What services and kind of care can you and your relative expect?

- What notice must be given on either side?

- Is a full assessment undertaken before approval?

Once you have made the decision on a care home being right for you and your loved one, you can think about how to make it homely. A good dementia home may have memory boxes outside bedrooms to help residents recognise the room as their own.

What happens now – the good care plan basics

I will now take you through the forms that make up the bulk of your loved one's care plan and the reasons for them.

Funding

This is a very complex subject with criteria that change all the time and are different in some counties. The best thing to do is contact your local authority or the CAB; sometimes care homes can also advise you. Top-ups and limits also depend on a person's individual circumstances and the care home's fees.

Pre-assessment

Pre-assessment is when a care manager will come to see your loved one, assess their health and capabilities to make sure the home can meet their needs and get some background information. Sometimes in cases where social funding is required a social worker will come out and do their own assessment; they will decide from this if your loved one needs care at home, residential care or nursing care.

The care plan

This is a massive folder you and your relative will be able to see on request at any time.

Probably the most important part is the 'contact details' section. This page provides your contact details and any other next of kin details. You should be asked if you are happy to be contacted day or night in the event of illness, falls, death.

If there are any complicated family dynamics or people your relative does not wish to see then the home will need to know so all staff on the floor can be made aware of this.

A life map

This is a map showing your loved one's past, achievements, hobbies, occupation etc. This will also note likes, dislikes and any routines that they have. This information is very important; it gives all staff a chance to get to know the resident's history and what they like to talk about or spend their time doing.

Health checks

These few checks are often done by senior carers or nurses. They will normally consist of blood pressure check, oxygen reading, temperature reading and urine sample test. These checks do two things; firstly, they give us a baseline, so if your relative is poorly we can compare readings to check for any concerns and contact a GP if needed. Secondly, they let us know if there are any abnormalities present on admission that we should check with a GP.

A photo consent form may need to be signed giving permission for nursing staff to take pictures of any skin concerns and also a face photo for medication rounds; this helps with drug administration safety. Where there are any skin injury concerns a photo gives us the chance to look back to make sure conditions are healing correctly. Any drug or food allergies will be noted, along with what medication the patient is on and when this was last reviewed.

Laundry tagging and valuables inventory

All clothes should be tagged with a name. Most homes now provide netting washing bags with a number tag sewn on to prevent missing clothing. In many homes a list will be made of every item brought in and any valuables will be photographed for insurance purposes.

Mobility assessment

This is essential for any care setting to have for a resident's safety and comfort as well as the staff's. This gives all staff information on what aids need to be used for each transfer, chair to bed, chair to wheelchair etc. If there is any uncertainty on the correct ways then a physio may be called in for advice.

Safety

Safety for people who wander more

In too many homes I have seen carers constantly sitting people down, saying 'you will fall'. Years ago I looked after a lady who had been transferred from another home where they had prescribed her sleeping medication because they said that if she was sleepy she did not wander so much, yet these drugs make people more likely to fall. A good home will have pressure pads: alarmed mats that when they are walked over just alert staff that residents are on the move, not to go and stop them walking. Seat alarms will go off once a resident's weight is taken off a seat as well.

Discouraging mobility will cause patients to lose the use of their limbs more quickly, which in turn will make hoists needed. A good home will encourage people to do what they can to keep their independence.

Bed safety

More and more homes avoid bed rails where possible due to the entrapment risk. This said, if your loved one wants or is used to bed rails, or if they say they are epileptic and could have a seizure at any time and fall out of bed, then staff should be happy to provide them with a risk assessment in place. Anyone who has bed rails with padding on should be on hourly checks to make sure they are safe; these checks are recorded by a form that should be in their room and signed every hour. Low beds and crash mats are sometimes nicer options. These are beds very low to the floor and large padded mats that look like gym mats on either side so in the event of a fall damage is minimised. All residents in any care setting should be regularly checked on throughout the night as well as the daytime.

Safety of staff looking after residents

Sadly I have worked with various people in my career who have been taking things they should not have been, which affected their attitude. Some even turned up for work drunk, experiencing mood swings, paranoia etc. While I was of the mind that we needed to get these staff help should they want to stay in the job, it soon became apparent that management was not overly concerned about acting because this was not taking place in our building. At one understaffed home a carer showed up drunk and the manager's response was, 'Well, at least it's another pair of hands.' Great, I thought, and if someone has an accident, as it is only a residential home, how will this look to paramedics? I know that I will never again be put in this position where residents are at risk, but how many other homes have staff with these habits?

Health and behaviour

Continence and bowels

While I am sorry to have to be so personal these are an important part of general overall health in everyone. If people are often experiencing the embarrassment of incontinence episodes, and regular toileting trips do not alleviate the problem, action should be taken. In these cases a continence assessment for your loved one can be filled out and sent off to see if pads can be obtained on the NHS. While soiled clothes are of no concern to good care staff, the dignity of this person is being affected, so action should be taken.

It is worth noting if patients are all put in pads. My current care home's policy is to have regular staff to assist with toileting to avoid pads if possible; this, however, is one of only a couple of places I have seen this good plan in practice.

Your loved one should have a bowel chart; this will show pictures of motions so staff can see what is normal routine, colour, form etc. This means that if there are any changes, staff will seek advice from nurses to see if it warrants a doctor's advice.

Skin integrity

By observing skin changes and acting on them, pressure areas can be prevented. Again pictures of any concerns will be taken so that we can see if an area is not improving, in which case we can involve tissue viability nurses or dermatology for expert advice.

Where people have issues with mobility or have skin issues already they will often be assessed to see if they need pressure-relieving mattresses. The airflow moves each ridge in the bed to alleviate pressure on each body part. Some people will need to have their position changed for them every two to four hours as well; there should be a form that is filled in at each time with their new position, the date and time, and the signatures of the two people attending.

A warning on having bed care only

Residents in care should be encouraged to get up into a comfy chair in their room, sit in the lounges with others etc. Airflow cushions for chairs and wheelchairs are available, and for this reason your loved one should not be left in bed every day. They can be up and about like any other residents unless they choose not to. Special recliners as well as adapted wheelchairs are giving more and more people quality of life. Good care homes will not condemn someone to bed 24/7 but will look into the possibility of getting them out and supporting their quality of life.

Must score

What can I say; all we see lately are failures in nutrition and hydration needs, people dehydrated and malnourished. In my 'concerns' section later I explain how I have witnessed these goings-on. The malnutrition universal screening tool is a precious chart in a good care setting. This chart helps us to work out for each patient what their risk is for malnourishment.

As your new home does not know your loved one, even if they are not in an at-risk group it is advisable for staff to fill in a food and fluid chart for a week just to check on their intake. By seeing what is offered and refused, staff will also learn what types of foods and drink your loved one is really enjoying. I have had people who have a sweet tooth and mainly eat cake or other puddings; so what? No, it is not the nutritious ideal, but it is their choice; staff can encourage, not force.

Freshly-made soups and puddings can be made with cream to support calorific intake. At my first home food was mainly made from scratch, no tinned or packet puddings etc. If staff still feel the right nutrients are not being taken then they should seek advice from a dietician or GP about build-up drinks if needed. Fluid intake is a big concern with the elderly. With a little thought jellies, ice creams, soup and yoghurts can all be included in daily intakes.

I have had a relative say in front of his dad, 'Can't you send him into hospital for a drip?' His dad had decided he would not eat and drink because he wanted to die. This is why it is also important that care homes audit all the charts so if there are any concerns we can act on them. If you come in to see your relative for lunch, or at coffee time, it may encourage them to eat/drink.

At the end of the day it is important that residents in a home have access to fluids and food whenever they want them, and that there are enough care staff available to help people who are unable to take food or fluids independently.

Behavioural charts

I can hear your gasp at this expression. Basically at times of distressed behaviours or verbal/physical aggression these charts may be used. These charts tell us what was happening around the resident at the time of the behaviour, how it was dealt with and what we feel could be done to prevent the situation from occurring again. If we are unable to alleviate these behaviours then these charts are kept to show any other teams that become involved in that resident's care. With all the best will in the world, there are times when techniques such as distraction just don't help. Sometimes there may be signs of withdrawal and lack of interest, and any signs like these may suggest to us that a resident needs help from a professional in the mental health field to get through these feelings.

Speech and swallowing

Many people in care have suffered from strokes which have caused speech and language problems and weakness. This can also cause swallowing difficulties, so it may be important to assess your relative's swallowing reflexes. If some food textures cause coughing then your loved one could be at risk from aspiration, inhaling food into the lungs, and this in turn can cause pneumonia. Speech and language therapists can give advice to staff and relatives on meal times.

General appearance requirements

Just being older does not mean that people do not like to look nice. If your loved one likes help with makeup, painted nails etc. then this care should still be continued in a care setting. Glasses and hearing aids are very important, but so are chiropody treatments and hairdresser visits. All the things they liked at home should continue wherever your loved one is.

Mental wellbeing

Boredom and lack of stimulation in homes is like mental torture, and often I have seen how people with dementia enjoy simple things like a rummage box, a pencil and notepad, tape measure and bit of string. Such small things can go a long way, but will a patient be allowed to have them? Health and safety has gone mad, so let's explore why. Surely giving someone a cloth for dusting or letting them help lay tables gives them a purpose and makes them feel useful. Let's take the example of a bedroom rug or a pressure mat in bedrooms: these need a risk assessment to be approved. Even hot water bottles or a resident wishing to keep alcohol in a room has to have paperwork attached. Should people in wheelchairs have to wear seatbelts? This can be seen as restraint, yet if they were to tip out without one would this mean we had neglected their safety? Everything really is paperwork, yet the end result, making someone feel their life is not worthless, is priceless.

Another stupid thing: many patients have kissed me on the cheek after I have tucked them into bed, and one day, when my resident was upset and reached out to me for a hug, I was told not to respond because this was seen as inappropriate behaviour. How can someone in the caring profession who actually cares ignore a cry for help like this – be so cold? 'Just tell them it will all be OK and walk away,' I was told. 'They are our wages, not friends.' I could not bear the thought of this happening to any of my relatives. The hierarchy of needs should be taught to some of my past managers who call themselves caring managers, because many basic needs were not being met.

Capacity and best interests

Now for a very tricky and complex subject that will not necessarily affect your loved one at all. If a patient's decisions are causing any concerns for their safety and welfare, or if they are making unsafe requests, then health professionals may talk to you about having a capacity assessment carried out. The Mental Capacity Act and Deprivation of Liberty Safeguards (MCA DOLS) has been in force since 2005 and this provides a legal framework which is there to stop unlawful deprivation of liberties occurring. All vulnerable people in care or hospitals who have been assessed to lack the capacity to make their own decisions are protected from harm. It can be the Primary Care Trust (PCT) care and hospital settings that have responsibility for applying this act. Full details can be obtained from a care home manager or the CAB. These acts are sometimes short-term to protect people, for example, while they are recovering from a brain injury and unable to make decisions safely. These actions are never taken lightly but are taken out of a duty of care to your loved ones.

End-of-life planning

One of the hardest parts to discuss for anyone, yet the most important part to get right. The main aim of an end-of-life plan is to have things already in place for when the time arrives. It is crucial to discuss whether you and your loved one want a Do Not Resuscitate order in place, for example; if you do, you and the GP will need to sign a form after a proper discussion on how the order will work. Also important is your loved one's choice in care; if they were to become very poorly, would they want to stay in the care home rather than be sent to hospital? Many people are of the mindset that if there is nothing hospital can provide for comfort that their care home can't, they would rather be where they know the staff and are in their own surroundings. You should be asked if there are any requests such as a priest visiting near the end, any cultural beliefs that need to be followed and whether you have an undertaker of your own choice you would like used.

These choices and requests are personal to everyone; there is no one right or wrong way. A good care home gives you support to achieve your needs, and all homes should have staff members trained in this area of expertise. There may be an opportunity to follow advanced care planning for someone, where you can discuss needs for the end of life. Sometimes, though, life takes us by surprise and a loved one gets sick very quickly, which leaves little time.

It may be that when you know your loved one is near passing you cannot face the shock and pain. Remembering them as they were is the better way for some people. Whatever your choice, this will be respected and you should be supported by staff. Some people need more professional support after losing a loved one and any care home will be able to advise you on people to contact for further support. Death is very personal for everyone and all staff should try to help your loved one achieve what is a good death in their eyes. Staff will discuss any interventions to prevent oral problems and any other common happenings at this time.

Ways of keeping your loved one as comfortable as possible

- If someone is unable to take medications orally then a GP may be contacted and permission may be requested for use of a syringe driver. This little contraption will be placed into a skin site and will administer medications at the rate and dosage set by the doctor. Various medications can be administered in this way such as morphine, for pain relief, and hyoscyamine, which is a medication that helps to dry up respiratory secretions if needed. Although patients are often very non-responsive when on drugs like these, they should not be suffering from pain and discomfort.

- Lip salve can be used in cases of dry and cracked lips and mouths, when fluid offered is not being taken and other medications may dry the mucosa, but so also can frozen cubes of tinned pineapple juice that are crushed before being placed on the tongue. There are oral gel sprays that can moisten the mouth for comfort too.

- Patients should be turned regularly to prevent marking of the skin, and staff should be monitoring closely for any changes or signs of discomfort. Often there is no output of urine or faeces when no food or fluid is being taken, although this should be checked on in case the patient needs changing at any time.

Signs that the time to say goodbye is near

People often ask, 'How long do you think it will be?' The sad truth is nobody can give a definite answer to you. I have known a man given a three-month prognosis to pass exactly three months later as the doctor had stated; however, a lovely man in my street who had prostate cancer was given six months, and he lived for just over five years. Some people go on for months and staff think 'any day now', but nine months later, hardly eating or drinking, they are still with us.

Shortly before death the patient's extremities (their nose, ear tips, hands and feet) may be cold and purple/blue, their breathing may change and you may hear staff say they are Cheyne–Stoking. Some people have a massive loose bowel action before passing, but everyone is different; some people may pass with none of these signs.

The guilt if they go and we are not there

Often people feel guilt that they were not in the room when their loved one passed, but this need not be the case. Sometimes I or families have sat with someone for hours, even days. Then you might leave the room for a few minutes for a drink or the toilet and on returning find they have passed on. In my mind this has led me to think: is it possible these patients are almost waiting to be alone before dying? In their own way, do they not want loved ones to actually watch them go? We will never know, I guess, but the thing is that without someone being constantly by their side 24/7 there is a possibility that this could happen. Death is a very personal thing for everyone; we all do what we think is right for us, and that is what matters.

After death

After your loved one has passed, sometimes next of kin will have to identify them. There is a possibility you will be asked to give permission for a post-mortem if the cause of death needs to be confirmed. However this can also be done without consent. Once this has been dealt with, the body will be kept in the chapel of rest until the funeral. Staff in the hospital or home will keep possessions safely until the person administering the estate comes to collect them, upon which a receipt should be given.

Keeping an eye on your loved one's care

Now that your loved one is settling in, it is normal to feel you want to make sure everything is as good as it seems. There is nothing wrong with this, and I have done it in the past when patients of mine have had to change homes.

- Pop in at different times of the day

- Take note of the menu on display; does the food being served match the menu, and does it look appetising and colourful?

- Book to have a meal with your relative. Are patients being encouraged to do what they can but fed tactfully and patiently if needed?

- Go in for elevenses with your relative; this is a good way of seeing that they are up, washed and dressed nicely and that their mid-morning drink is given.

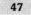

- If you are in the communal lounges, are the staff helping people with drink if needed? Are they moving anyone into comfy chairs? Note if they are speaking gently to patients and always keeping them informed on what they are doing as they are helping them. While staff are helping people to eat and drink, are they sitting at eye level? Being towered over by staff will make people feel intimidated.

- How do you see people being addressed: by their proper name or as 'sweetie', 'darling', 'poppet'? Being addressed with terms like these is a pet hate of many people, understandably. People being spoken to in a patronising tone as if they are a child is also unacceptable.

- Have you seen people knocking before entering rooms?

- Most patients will have some charts in their room with them, recording food, fluid, continence etc.; are these being filled in properly?

- In the bedroom should always be fresh drink and a glass. The en suite should have fresh towels and facecloths; the bins should be emptied regularly. The living space should all be nice and clean, with fresh bedding. Pull it back and check;

I do, and would do if it were my parents as well. If you find any grumbles let someone know; a good place will be glad you have pointed things out for their attention.

- If your loved one seems distant or not their usual self to you, always make time to find someone and make them aware of your concern.

Many people are lucky, having family who will visit them, but others not so. I remember feeling very sad when one of my ladies who had dementia had her birthday in December; the family lived 10 miles away and came to see her once a year. This lady had recently picked up one of the dementia weighted dolls; she would rock it on her knee, singing away, when staff would barely get a smile. The family went mad on seeing this, snatching it out of her arms, saying she was not a child; I remember the expression on her face to this day. This doll went to bed with her at night as well. I explained to her family that she had chosen to pick this doll up and not let it go; it was not forced upon her. She also had very few clothes, and the family were happy for her to have the clothes of people who had passed away. Seeing these things can make you appreciate everyone and everything that little bit more, but also makes us realise we need to be there for these people.

Hospital care concerns

There have been so many care failures within hospitals in the news lately, and sadly I have seen these myself.

I had a stage of having seizures and spent various times in A&E as well as on wards. My goodness, there are some staff who should not be in the job as well as many who are amazing. Here are a few of the things I witnessed:

- People on bedpans crying and ringing their bell to get off, nobody about. One lady was left on for over half an hour until I went to find someone.

- Food and drink left where patients cannot reach it, or patients otherwise going unfed. I have seen food dumped next to patients who are asleep and the full plate taken half an hour later from the still-sleeping patient.

- There was an elderly lady in the cubicle opposite me; she had come in the same time. Over the four-hour period we were there neither of us was offered a drink. She was confused and had bedrails up; I had to get someone to go to her as she was trying to climb them. It had been over two hours since someone had even checked on her; she could have died in this time and no one would have known.

- Dignity and hygiene: I have had to ask for bed rails to be cleaned of old blood, and to ask nurses to put gloves on when taking blood.

- The hierarchy: I once watched a young lady crying and vomiting with her curtains closed; her bell was going off and there were nurses just wandering. A sister peeped through the gap, saw she was vomiting and walked off. I heard her say to a healthcare assistant, 'Can you go to her next? It is your job.' In care we are a team working together; if a nurse is free, is it beneath her to fulfil someone's basic care needs?

I have had the pleasure to work with a few good staff. A nurse I worked with once said to me, 'Take note of patients who come out of hospital and how many of them have been catheterised. Many catheters are put in to avoid having to assist people to toilets, not for medical reasons.' She was right; many of those people left us being able to use the toilet with help. Another thing she pointed out, although more common for people with dementia, was the number of times sedating drugs have been newly prescribed when patients come out of hospital.

Too many care settings I have worked in seem to ask GPs whether they can administer things like Lorazepam PRN and other sedating drugs to a lot of patients. Rather than staff actually stimulating people who show frustration and finding other ways to help, they ask the nurse to give a pill as a first option. It is no wonder we have so many polypharmacy patients: patients on many medications. Carers do not think that every drug has a side effect, so we give another drug to counteract that one and they just increase. Teams in areas like mental health care are specialists in this field and I know if it were my mum or dad I would rather have an expert's opinion before getting out pills. Some previous care managers have said to me, 'It's not worth the paperwork trail; let's just get a GP to prescribe something.' Which is fine ... as long as they feel confident that no further professionals need to be informed. One thing I know is that I would rather do paperwork all day than have someone put on a potentially unnecessary drug. Don't get me wrong, these drugs are important to some and have their uses, but only when prescribed by the right professional in the right circumstances.

GPs can also have their issues. Now, I am very lucky, having a wonderful, kind GP who listens and cares; they have seen to residents of mine as well. However in my time I have been upset to come across GPs who see older people simply as people who don't have long anyway. I remember early on in my care days when an out-of-hours GP came out to see my very poorly patient and said they were too near the end to waste medication on. It left me wondering whether he would still have made this comment if the family had been with me. Surely anything to alleviate suffering, irrespective of how long they have left, is the patient's right, and surely it is a GP's job to administer this. We have so many wonderful caring doctors, but sadly there are a minority who should not, in my opinion, be practising with such a cold attitude.

Nursing staff and doctors are under immense pressure on all wards, and in both hospitals and care homes the ratios required for patient safety are unrealistic. So many managers giving direction on what needs to be improved, but no resources given to achieve this. So many more people going through A&E needing help, and all you hear about are staff and bed shortages. Staff working long shifts with little support. There seems to be the budget there to pay many senior managers to do one job while budgets for front-line staffing levels are cut back. My feeling is that while this continues we are at a stalemate. If wards are not given the staff to meet patients' needs, we will only continue to see an increase of complaints and failings surrounding standards of care in hospitals. For goodness' sake, last time I had blood taken my husband looked on in horror as they had to tie a rubber glove around my arm, having been unable to find a tourniquet; my friend's mum was given pillow cases to dry herself with because there were no towels. Doctors and nursing staff and HCAs are the ones on the floors of wards and care homes; when they need essential equipment, they should get it. We were on our last box of gloves in one care home because the budget had only allowed the order late. Not following basic infection control procedures poses a serious risk to patients and staff.

National standards in care settings – what to expect as a patient

You should be involved in your care and treatment options, supported and told what is happening at every stage

- You will be spoken with about your treatment, care and support. There will be support to help you make decisions and staff will respect your privacy and dignity.

- You will be given opportunities, support and encouragement to help you live as independently as possible.

- Before you receive any examination, care or treatment you will be asked if you agree or not.

You should expect care, treatment and support that meets your needs

- Your personal needs will be assessed to make sure you receive appropriate safe care that supports your rights.

- You will get the care that you and your professionals both agree will make the difference to your health and wellbeing.

- You will get the food and drink required to meet your dietary needs.

- You will receive co-ordinated care if you have more than one care provider or move between services.

- You can expect your care home to meet all your needs; for example, needs relating to culture, language, background, gender, disability, age, sexuality, beliefs.

You should expect to be safe

- You will be protected from abuse and risk of abuse.

- Staff will protect your human rights.

- You will have your medication given when needed in a safe way.

- You will be cared for in a safe, accessible place.

- You will not be harmed by unsafe or unsuitable equipment.

- You will be cared for in a clean environment where you are protected from infections.

You should expect to be cared for by staff with the right skills to do their job properly

- You will be cared for by staff who have the knowledge, experience and skills required to meet your health and welfare needs.

- There will always be enough members of staff available to keep you safe and meet your needs.

- You will be looked after by staff who are well managed and who have the chance to develop and improve their skills.

You should expect your care provider to routinely check the quality of their services

- Your care home provider will monitor the quality of their services to make sure they are safe.

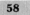

- Your personal and medical records/reports will be kept accurate, safe and confidential.

- You or someone acting on your behalf can complain and will be listened to. Your complaint will be acted on properly.

What finding a good home has shown me

Apart from saving my career, because I had made the decision that if this care home was the same as the others I was giving up on the care industry, my new place of work proved to me and still does to this day that there is a way that works and excellent care is possible.

In my mind, when a care setting is getting a minimum of £900 a week per patient, how could good care not be expected or achieved? Paying this money you could stay in a five-star hotel, which in my mind this group of homes is like, and have your own private nurse.

At some places I have been before, the things mentioned below were commonly seen or even considered normal practice:

- Poor-quality food, mostly out of tins or packets. Bread and milk out of date but used anyway.

Meals such as muffin and chips, fish fingers and kids' spaghetti hoops three times a week. Being told to scrape the outside off a black burned cake and put custard on it. Many staff speaking to management, who claim to have seen no problem with this.

- Some care homes have little choice of activities, and even then only at limited times. Often people are still in bed at 11.30 waiting to be washed and then it is lunch time, and therefore they miss out.

- Poor staff ratios. Now every home has true sickness leave and holidays, but when people were sick we often were told not to cover it, not to even try. I was lucky to be one of seven looking after a home of 43 residents, and many of these were dementia or nursing needs patients. Just two cleaners to clean many rooms and communal areas and to do laundry.

- Unreliable staff, and staff who were only doing the job for a wage. Family members arguing and working the same shifts. Staff who, when they were taking sick leave, posted on social networking sites that they were out and drunk. The manager said, 'Oh, they are young,' but my feelings are that these people rely on us.

- Being criticised by managers who work Monday–Friday 9–5 and do not come in when they are needed even when desperately short of staff. Being told rooms need to be filled quicker and budgets cut back because there are too many staff when we cannot cope with the residents we have.

- Being ignored by the big bosses. In some homes I have never seen a regional manager or director greet staff or speak to any residents as they walk past, not even a hello. It costs nothing to be polite and show an interest in making sure the people paying your wages are happy with their care.

Why I would not want to leave my new position

It has taken me 16 years to find a place that cares and holds my view that we can never have too-high standards when caring for people's loved ones. To find a place where the manager and deputy really care; where they spend time taking residents out, even. To find a place where it is clear that they have a true passion for good care; it is not just the wages.

These are the conditions I have always wanted to have in a home, but rarely before now have I seen these provided, and I think they are essential in care.

- I am on the highest wage for care I have ever been on – but I have always done this for the love, not the wage packet. Many homes still only pay minimum wage.

- Management and deputies support their staff and help on the floor, rather than staying in the office.

- Big bosses speak to staff and residents about care.

- We have regular supervision to check we are giving the best we can to our patients.

- Concerns are acted on and dealt with; there is no favouritism in the ranks.

- Where there are real concerns the correct disciplinary procedures are carried out if warranted.

- Never before have I had the pleasure of working in a home that offers a daily three-course breakfast. The residents here enjoy fresh food with homemade soups, puddings etc. rather than the basic brand of everything, which many homes use for cheapness.

- Management recognises the need for good staffing ratios to meet residents' needs.

- Staff that care: I can put my hand on my heart and say that every person I work with now would give care to any resident as if it were their own mum or dad.

The philosophies in care I believe in and stand by

Every person I care for is treated as if they were my own dearly loved mum or dad.

I have every respect for people who have ever blown the whistle, and always will. They are protecting the patients who are relying on staff for safe loving care and upholding the trust placed in us by loved ones of patients.

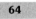

If you can cope with urine, faeces, sick, blood, false teeth and death, and if you can cope with getting the odd slap and abusive word from people, and if you can tell people the same thing 100 times an hour and still have a calm aura and sense of humour, then this is the best job in the world in my opinion. Care is not just coffee, cake and nice walks with patients, but what I can tell you is that to me this job is satisfying, rewarding and positive. It is making a difference to these people's lives, and I feel honoured to be part of this process.

True person-centred care – what is it and is it always given?

It infuriates me when people complain that homes have no set routine or structure, but guess what: this can be a good thing, and here is why. A true person-centred home works around residents' needs. It is fair enough that set mealtimes have their place, a care home needs to work around chefs; however, in places I have worked before, rules have often been 'breakfast 8–9 am, lunch 1 pm, supper 5 pm'. Now, being for the first time at a home where people's needs are worked around on a daily basis is lovely, but it is worrying to think back on all the false promises offered by so many out there. After all, every day is different; one day someone wants to get up at 4 am, another not until lunch. It is fair enough, like I say, for the set main meals, but why have some previously top-rated care homes said that if meals are not taken at these times the residents' only choice is biscuits? The moaning I heard if I went in and asked for toast because someone didn't want to get up for breakfast before 10 am; apparently the kitchen staff had plenty of time to sit outside with other staff after already having their break but weren't prepared to whip up some toast or an omelette. People requesting fresh fruit salad were told it was too expensive; only tinned fruit and frozen meat and veg were allowed to be bought; portions were cut back, staff levels cut back, and then, lo and behold, managers got a pay rise and a new car. Patients were suffering from the cutbacks, as were staff, but this was seen as acceptable.

It is wrong to expect any resident to work around the times that suit us, so any structure should fit around their choices for the day rather than being dictated by managers. Homes need to ask themselves: are they doing right by their residents or just doing what's easiest for them?

In my opinion, although every home up until now has said they are person-centred, only now do I see true person-centred care happening. I am in the only home I have ever worked where showers are offered 24/7. Some patients get up at 4 am and request a shower; I wake at 5 am and shower, so why shouldn't they be able to? The home they are in is now theirs and they should be able to choose to bathe, shower or wash when they want to. I bet you are thinking now that your own place would never allow enough staff to be on the floor for this to be a reality; this should not be the case, though, should it?

Activities – ideal for some, not for everyone

At my home we have outings, cheese and wine evenings, take-away nights and many trips out. Not everyone wants to participate, though. Some people never did these sorts of things at home and sat in front of the telly all day; if this is their wish, then fine. I had a chap who never left his room; he said to me on admission that he had led a solitary life and did not like people. Fair enough, I said, but I always gave him a choice and told him what activities were on. He never left his room until he died; he watched DVDs in his room and had wine and chocolates that he had bought, but this was the ideal life for him and it was his choice. We would always have a giggle and would talk of our love for animals; he said animals were better than people and he thought I had been a horse in my previous life because I have very long hair, which he said was like a horse's tail plaited.

Along the way we meet many different people, all with different backgrounds and personalities. All staff should get to know people well – their character, their needs, their beliefs – because coming into a home does not mean it all stops. This is their identity and they should never lose this as it is an important part of their life.

Behind closed doors – a crisis that needs to be changed

So many people in the news have expressed concerns about how particular care homes seemed so good.

I have been sucked in, as are many others. A care home may sound amazing in the beginning, but failings can soon become apparent.

I have been in the position where there have been failings and, had it not been for a colleague, I would have been next in line to whistle-blow. Some people say to me, 'But why did you stay so long?' But you do, because you worry about the residents and you think to yourself about what will happen if you are not there; what if it were your mum or dad? There would be times at some homes when I would look on a shift and think, *Oh no, that staff mix*; so many people there were concerned, yet nothing was done. Recently a care home was inspected and the inspection found that staff were asked by management not to report any concerns to anyone except within work, which is very wrong. In previous places I have been at, many times I have reported various concerns – even beyond management, in some homes – but nobody cared.

A lady who has now sadly passed away used to come and visit a very elderly gentleman I cared for a while ago. Many times she raised her own concerns over a care home and nothing was done with her reports. Sadly, having experienced failures in the system through work, I can see how frustrated she must have been in her fight. It amazes me how on inspections patients have said, 'Oh, I won't complain' out of fear; it also has amazed me when inspectors have not spoken to residents who are capable of giving opinions, making their own judgements. This lady was furious when, not long after she expressed her concerns, the care home in question had a report and passed with flying colours; luckily it has changed hands and now, I am told, is much improved.

Now, I know for a fact that had a few of the homes I worked at had 24-hour CCTV in bedrooms, lounges and dining areas – had they seen the poor care, the quality of the food, the staff on mobile phones – then these problems would have been addressed.

People may say that CCTV is an invasion of privacy, of our rights etc., but relatives have often said that they wish there were cameras in care homes and I have to agree. I would be happy to be watched, as I am sure many others would; why would we object if we are doing the job properly? What scares me, though, is the question of what we might see from many homes if they had CCTV installed, and what percentage of those homes have just had glowing reports?

Many inspectors, as they are from a medical background, might know the home manager because of their nursing qualifications. There should be no link between these two people, because this leaves room for reports that are glowing when there are problems; this in turn, in my opinion, could put residents at risk. Many news stories lately have talked about errors by professionals; abuse cases in our region doubled this year. These news stories, I am afraid, are the tip of the iceberg, and this scares me and many others out there who will one day need care for their relatives. We need transparency in all reports on findings.

I've heard some wonderful news recently: families and carers are to do care home inspections with inspectors. Great, there will be no shortage of takers for this one, and many of the homes I have experienced should be shaking in their boots. Involvement in inspections like this is the only way carers will have a voice in many homes. I still have old acquaintances in many of my former homes who have been shocked and disheartened after inspections have found the homes compliant. Many of them fool themselves into thinking it will be OK; they just do their bit and go home, feeling intimidated into silence. Only a minority that I know of have ever spoken out. Carers should never feel afraid to speak; we have a duty of care to these people, after all. I find it so sad that families have had to prove abuse in many homes. How many more will suffer abuse before something really changes?

Horrible things that nurses and even managers have said to me over 16 years

My fingers are crossed that no person who reads these anecdotes feels that there is nothing wrong with them. If you do then my hope would be that

73

you step back and think about your role very hard, because all of these shout 'abuse' to me.

- One of my worst and most upsetting situations was where a manager told me to stop giving a patient drink. This dying man was too weak to drink off a spoon; he was taking water through a syringe and opening his mouth for more. She said it was abusive and force-feeding, that he would die soon anyway so I should stop. I would wait until she was not around and carry on. His family came in and did this for him because his lips were cracked and bleeding and he wanted the water. How could a nurse have this view on someone who was conscious and opening his mouth to swallow the water?

- Care manager: 'Don't take her down to the coffee morning; take the ones that can communicate and look better.'

- 'Why are you not giving this medication?' I was asked. 'You can't just say it was refused; it can be hidden.' Giving medication covertly is an offence and I was not prepared to take a person's rights away just to please staff. Hiding medication in a patient's food so they don't refuse it is just not something which can be done because we feel it is right; yet it is done, and in many homes. I used to get so sick of going into patients' rooms and seeing their pills left on the table or spat down their front, and yet all the pills were signed for. Until the medication has been witnessed as swallowed those sheets should not be signed; yet another case of legal documents not telling the truth, and many care managers didn't see the problem.

- Care manager: 'I don't see what the issue is; I would eat it.' This was in response to a cold meal. Many residents complained but, again, nothing was done. £200 was seen as plenty to feed 51 residents for a week. To have healthy meals and fresh fruit for my family of five we spend nearly this.

- After reporting blood in a catheter to a nurse I was told, 'None of us on this weekend can change the catheter; it can wait until Monday. You're only a carer, so don't worry about it.'

- Something that angers me to this day: when (again) we were working with unsafe staffing levels, it took us a while to answer a call bell and when we got there a nurse stood at the door, scowling. She said, 'The bell has been ringing for over ten minutes and this person has been incontinent.' This little elderly frail man was covered in faeces. 'It is your job,' she said, and she left. Now, in those ten minutes she could have dealt with his discomfort, but instead she chose to stand around watching the call bell times. The unnecessary embarrassment this had caused the poor man, who was crying as we cleaned him up, was obvious. On speaking to a head nurse we were told that they are in dark blue for a reason and their job is not dealing with this type of care, which disgusts me.

- A very dangerous situation I have seen before is where nurses have been given a treatment by a GP and chosen not to give it to the patient for a few days to see how they go first. This is a dangerous situation for anyone. If a GP has prescribed a medication and it is not being administered, action can and should be taken. This is where the importance of documentation comes in; after a GP has been in, their advice should be noted with full instructions on how the medication should be given, when to start it etc. My poor experiences have left me hoping that these situations are not common practice. I hope there are care homes that will read this book and think that this is terrible and would never let it happen in their home.

- I have seen complete lack of respect for a patient who could not communicate. Early in my care days a matron of a care home had no choice but to help me clean someone. This lady had had several strokes previously and lost movement down one side and all speech; to me she spoke with her eyes, but to this matron she was nothing. While cleaning the matron said, 'God, this stinks; what has she been eating?' with no thought for her feelings. I actually remember saying there and then, 'How could you say that?' to which she replied, 'This woman knows nothing of what is said or done; she is not with it up there.' There were various things going on in that home, and early in my care days I felt overwhelmed by the way I was being taught. People who could not speak for themselves were woken up at 5 am and left dressed in a chair all day in this room; however, what this carer did not realise was that the lady who shared the room with this stroke patient was 'with it' enough to mention to her daughter-in-law that she was disturbed at five in the morning on some days. This carer still works there to this day, nothing done about it, and this home has had other issues since.

- Another example of complete lack of respect was a home where I actually visited a patient who I had looked after before. When I popped in it was lunch time; he was in a dining room full of patients and a nurse came in and just lifted his shirt to administer his insulin. She did not even speak to him and say what was coming, no thought for his privacy or dignity whatsoever. I have worked in homes that use patients' prescribed pads for other residents: theft, basically. I have seen homes where pads were broken into two so they lasted longer and the other half given to different patients. It is horrendous and despicable. Because pads provided by the NHS often have a daily allocation of four over a 24-hour period, this was a care home's answer. Had these residents been supported and prompted with toileting many of them would not have had a need for pads, but attempts to convince carers who did not care to help with this fell on deaf ears.

- Finally, the advice given to me by a manager who specialised in end-of-life care: 'Pull yourself together; if you feel hurt after death you are emotionally attached. Let's concentrate on getting the room emptied and refilled again. If you were professional like myself you would feel nothing. They are just another number, and this is God's waiting room; they come in one door and out another.' This was the speech that tipped my feelings on the poor care out there, and it is why I am writing this book. The day I can feel like that is the day I will resign from care.

Now, if this is what managers and trained nursing staff are practising, what hope have new staff got of learning the right way to protect our future loved ones? We should be teaching good care practice.

Too many homes – same attitude from staff

People would be horrified if they knew what often goes on in care homes, and I want it to stop. Bedclothes changed sometimes once a month; I once commented on a stained bed and a carer said it was only a small wee stain. I would not have slept on it or expected my parents to either. Charts falsified, which managers in my past have been made aware of; I have known for a fact people have not eaten or drunk what is recorded on their intake charts. Pathetic food portions; at some homes in which I have worked the chef did not like doing different meals for diabetics, so instead only diabetic puddings were made and everyone had to have these puddings and cakes, which of course did not meet all dietary needs. People sitting in lounges with walking aids left out of reach so they don't get up, call bells that seem to have magically unplugged themselves overnight and some patients not given drinks after 5 pm to stop them needing the loo at night. Carers taking no notice of handling reports; they cannot be bothered with the hoist and so are lifting people under the arms, risking their patient because this move has the potential to dislocate the patient's shoulder and the lifter's back.

The importance of dignity

Many a time I have had to tell other staff to think about what is wrong in the situation we are in. When I have new carers and they go to wash someone on the bed, leaving their whole body exposed, I ask them to consider how they would feel if they were the one being washed. Whatever part being washed should be the only part visible. Staff should knock on doors rather than just barging in. When residents need the toilet, they should always be asked if they would like to be given the call bell and left in privacy.

Care companies, managers and their expectations of staff

Firstly, I will say there is NO excuse for any abuse of any kind.

Some companies I have worked for previously have had the following expectations of staff, which are not safe and unrealistic:

- Minimum wage for care staff.

- Minimum holiday legally possible given.

- Unpaid breaks; often staff do not even get these due to lack of workers.

- No support from management.

- Little training or supervision.

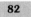

- Pressure to get rooms filled and money in without the resources to cope with residents' needs.

- Lack of opportunity for staff to have their say.

On top of all the other demands expected of carers, poor working conditions like these make stressed staff, which in turn means poorly staff because they are overstretched. This can lead to tense feelings which may rub off onto the residents' care.

The big mistake made by many companies is expecting carers to be responsible not just for personal care, but for preparing food, washing up, laundry and cleaning. This is not safe or hygienic. Too many companies seem to think that they can save money by giving carers all these duties, and I have been in many homes where they are expected of you. This often leaves staff who already have to cope with minimal staff-to-patient ratios struggling to give even basic care for residents. Do I think that it is acceptable to help someone who has been doubly incontinent, then change my polythene pinny to a different-coloured one to go and prepare food or wash up? No, I do not. We cannot be kitchen assistants, carers and laundry staff and still be able to look after residents. This is not how I would want my mum or dad looked after if I were paying all that money, not by a long shot.

I have felt many a time in previous homes that there are times management needs to actually work the floor as carers. Some managers don't even come onto the floor, which is completely unacceptable. Some are quite happy to sit listening in their office, ignorant of their patients' needs and wellbeing, as call bells continue for a long time, and may even walk past the room which is ringing without popping their head around the door to check the patient is not on the floor or in danger.

I worked once with a good carer who told me some harrowing tales of how her previous company had worked. Members of staff who had had their final warnings or disciplinary action for repeated poor care got called into the office for the ultimatum: 'Hand in your notice and we will give a good reference, otherwise we will sack you and give you a poor one.' This meant many people were going to another home where they would possibly put residents at risk because their new employer had a good reference for them.

Now every time I have changed care jobs I have been told, 'Our home is different; we are driven by

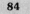

person-centred care before money and numbers.' I am now on the eighth home, and this is one of the few that have stayed true to their word. Every person here loves our residents like their own and puts the residents first, which is how it should be. For the first time I love going into work and feel proud to be part of such a good company. At the end of the day, the whole team has worked so hard for our residents and I know whoever is coming on the next shift is going to give care as loving as ours.

Supporting your staff to raise care standards

As a manager, you have one of the most important job roles: making sure every resident is protected from harm, respected and valued for who they are.

I hope my views from the front line will mould the way others think when giving care, improving the safety of staff and patients.

My home is the way it is today because the management have built it up and sustain it with high standards. Your home is as good as your care team, and if you take care of them your home should have a good reputation for care.

Together we must rebuild faith and trust in the care sector, for the sake of the people out there needing to place loved ones into care.

- Make sure there are enough staff to meet residents' needs. This is an important area to budget more on. People who look around want to see that needs can be met.

- Make sure staff get their breaks.

- Give all your staff support; let them know your door is open for concerns and they will be listened to.

- Praise staff regularly; a 'thank you' means so much more in this job.

- Give opportunities for staff meetings.

- If problems arise, deal with staff appropriately and with no favouritism.

- Be mindful if employing relatives of employees.

- Most importantly, once in a while go up on the floor, see what is going on. Do you have enough care staff to provide for residents' needs? Speak to the residents; do they seem happy with the care they have had today? Sometimes we can learn in this way about things that should be changed, what may work better etc. This will also earn you respect. Some people don't like seeing the manager on the floor, but it is an important part of their care role to check on care standards, and not just from their office.

Training and its importance

I am going to list just the basic training that I feel should be mandatory for everyone working in this area, to protect ourselves and the safety of people's loved ones.

- Deprivation of Liberty and Capacity Act/best interests training. With laws changing often, it is very important that staff understand the meaning of these laws and how and when we may need to consider evaluating a resident's ability to make decisions.

- Fire safety training. Everyone should know what they must do upon spotting a fire or hearing the fire alarms; everyone should know the fire zones and evacuation procedures. Should this become a reality rather than a practice, everyone must be able to exit the building safely.

- First aid training. Everyone should have basic training for what to do if they walk into a room to find someone on the floor or not breathing. The seconds spent waiting for nurses or paramedics can make all the difference. Another essential point, however: **are all staff aware of who has a DNR order in place?**

- Anaphylaxis recognition, perhaps caused by medication side effects, food allergies, flu jabs being given in care settings: all staff should know what the symptoms are and how to act.

- Health and safety training. Do staff know where the policy is, who is responsible for what, who to report things to?

- Manual handling training. All staff should have proof of this training before starting in a care setting and using equipment.

- End of life/dealing with death training. Helping staff to cope with complex needs, syringe drivers, preparing the body etc. Staff should know what to look for in the end stages and support each other as well as the family. Not everyone drifts off quietly and some deaths can be very traumatic.

- Catheter and continence care. Staff should know how to care properly for catheters, how they should be sited, how to recognise blockages/urinary retention and infection sites etc.

- Dementia care and behaviours that challenge. Staff need to understand complex behaviours and how to deal with them and document if needed. We should also look at other ways we can overcome these if possible before we resort to medications, unless specialists advise them.

- Safeguarding. This is one of the biggest concerns in care lately: keeping your patients safe, recognising abuse and reporting.

- Whistle-blowing. These policies can vary between homes and areas. If you listen and act on staff concerns then they may not need to go further; however, anyone has the right to talk over concerns with the CQC if they have good reason for bypassing senior line staff.

- Pressure area awareness. All care staff should know the basics on how pressure sores can happen, what to look for, grades of pressure areas and treatments. As with most things, though, prevention is better than cure.

- Nutrition and hydration training, another area very prominent in the press lately due to failures. Staff should understand the importance of good nutrition and hydration, ways we can improve intake safely, and actions to take if people are losing weight or failing to eat or drink.

- Control of substances hazardous to health. In care homes there will be many chemicals we may come into contact with. It is helpful for care staff to have a basic understanding of the importance of this area.

- Infection prevention/control. All staff in this environment are exposed to bodily fluids and care settings can quickly develop a case of norovirus that spreads, so barrier nursing training and basic control procedures should be taught to all in contact with patients. Staff should be aware of the correct bins/colour-coded bags to use for clinical waste, sharps etc.

- Basic food hygiene. At some point all staff will provide food and drinks, possibly reheating food. Temperatures, food storage, hand washing etc. should all be taken on board by staff.

- Reporting and record keeping. The importance of all the documentation should be explained. Staff look at me even now in horror when I say that a chart is a legal document and could be used in a court of law if there were to be a dispute on care given. If it is not written, it did not happen.

- Caldicott principles. Everyone should be aware of the six principles and their meaning and importance.

- Dignity in care. Staff should understand the importance of dignity and privacy when looking after the private and personal care of patients.

There are many more truly interesting courses out there, but these in my view are basic ones that cover areas all carers have to deal with on a daily basis in their job.

Staffing

This is the biggest problem in care homes. When I was one of just two members of staff for 20 residents – which I feel is unsafe and unfair, although all too often normal – I would think of the time-related issues that these shortages created.

Take washing as an example. Washing or bathing someone properly takes a good half an hour, and some people need two carers for hoisting, washing etc. Breakfast would be from 8 am; this took an hour for two of us, sometimes more. So we would often be left with just two and a half hours for the two of us to wash 20 people before lunchtime at 12 noon. Management knew we struggled and told us these were acceptable numbers for what the budget allowed. This left each resident, on average, 7.5

minutes of our time for washing, when they were paying £1,000 a week; it doesn't say this in the posh brochures, does it?

This is why, when you are looking for a home, asking how many carers are on is important. Don't just ask the manager, though; ask yourself how many carers you have seen, because what the manager says and the reality can be different.

I would not expect my mum or dad to get 7.5 minutes to be properly washed, nor would I expect them to still be in bed at noon, but that is what happens in too many places; if they don't have enough staff to get everyone up in the morning, they leave the ones who can't complain till last. This is why, in my opinion, the CQC no longer having to insist on a certain staff ratio all the time leaves homes open to unacceptable care.

One thing I would love to see is volunteers who know the job and good care going in to maybe do a bit of volunteer work in care homes, spend one-on-one time talking to residents etc. I think this could make a real difference.

Appropriate appearance and behaviour

As a manager, one thing you need to be clear on is uniform and appearance amongst staff. In the past, I have been given a uniform policy which was never followed up on; staff did what they liked because they knew management would not act.

When people come to look at a home they look at staff and their appearance as well as managers. If people really care about the job, they will follow the policies.

- Most homes' policies state for health and safety reasons that ideally no items of jewellery apart from one stud in each ear and one plain wedding ring should be visible; all others should be covered or removed.

Dyed and garish hairstyles are usually not preferred; tattoos should be ideally covered where possible.

Nails should be short for safety; at one place I have worked it was common to see staff with false nails, which risked skin tears.

Appearance is not the only area in which policies must be enforced, of course. I once worked in a home where staff were warned ineffectually for months about texting on mobile phones at work, even in residents' rooms. We had a sign up saying that mobile phones were to go in lockers, but nothing was done to enforce it. People would text on corridor corners, which is so unprofessional. Sadly, I have heard of this in other homes, and I feel behaviour like this is unacceptable when we are giving personal care.

Smoking can also become an issue. While it is wrong to discriminate and it is the smoker's choice to smoke, there is nothing worse for patients than the smell of smoke when we are in close contact with them. All staff should have to change out of uniform to smoke, and the staff smoking area should not visible to visitors. At the moment many smoking areas are in visitors' car parks, and in a couple of my previous homes the chef was allowed to smoke outside in uniform. This looks so unhygienic.

The behaviour of your staff outside the home could also be a potential pitfall; people need to realise where their boundaries are. For example, they must understand that certain details about the company or residents should not be discussed on social networking sites.

The day and night shift divide

One of the biggest issues I come across is conflict between day and night staff, the moaning about who is out of bed in the mornings or still up at night. In too many homes I have witnessed these quibbles. Now these are effectively people's homes we are working in, yet staff are running around trying to get a certain number of residents up and so many into bed for night staff. At previous homes I became sick of staff saying that a particular resident was still up, or that they were not out of bed and dressed. Where is the 'person-centred' care that every home claims to provide?

The idea is that we are giving care 24 hours a day, 7 days a week. There are times when residents may want to stay up later or get out of bed at a different time. These waking times should not be dictated for staff's ease of work; these residents are paying for the privilege to choose what they want and when. Staffing levels should be at the point where nobody will be kept waiting for hours if they request to get up or go to bed. Obviously in this work we will come across people who are unable to express these wishes verbally, and so we have to judge if they seem tired, keep an eye out to see if they are in bed early but lie awake for a long time etc. This is why, where possible, having a rough guide of the routine they are used to may help. Members of staff who are dictating who they wish to have up or in bed at certain times can be seen as abusing their position, as this is taking away the residents' choices.

Identity theft

Sometimes care home staff are guilty of a sort of identity theft: stealing any sense of identity from residents by way of not seeing them for who they are.

Too many people I have seen in care homes are just lost as another number to have to look after. These people have had lives, been a mum, nan, auntie etc. and probably had a very good career; why are we failing to recognise everyone as individuals and talk about their lives? When working with few staff, when I did get my break I often would sit with a resident, looking at their photos and talking about their history. It is almost like most places just focus on why residents are in and what they can't do for themselves any more, rather than focusing on positives and on the fact that they still have lives to live.

I went on an end-of-life course a while ago where a Parkinson's nurse told us all that the average time spent in a care home before dying is two years. This certainly sounds upsetting, but all staff just need to make all the time every patient has as nice as possible. I detest going into care home lounges and seeing everyone asleep in a circle of wheelchairs in front of chat shows with people shouting abuse at each other; it's also common to see the television left on the kids' channels. Where are the nice old-fashioned films and news/documentary channels? There may of course be residents who genuinely like these programmes, which is different. This is why, as I have found with this home, having two lounges with tellies is good; this way every resident has a choice if they do not like one thing. Many care home residents also have tellies and even laptops in their rooms for when they want to sit quietly with their choice of programme. The ideal is that residents are supported to do what is possible to keep their minds active and care staff can help with this.

As a company you need to be clear on policies like these and be prepared to carry out any necessary follow-up for staff who do not take you seriously, for your residents' sake as well as your home's reputation. Staff need to know you are fair but will not be messed about with; after all, these staff are your future reputation on the line. A weak manager is a dangerous person to have responsibility for so many people's health and welfare.

It is a must to check occasionally on night staff; too many homes lately have caught them asleep with their feet up for hours rather than tending to residents. Do residents all have their call bells in reach and are they plugged in? With regular continence checks needed and paperwork to be updated, there should be plenty for staff to do. It is one thing for them to get their hourly break of the night, but staff taking themselves off for hours need to be seriously dealt with for the protection of your residents.

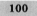

Staff demographics

Now, I have worked with a lovely male carer, but homes need to remember the importance of asking each resident if they are happy to be looked after by male or female staff. It is nice to have a male carer for the gentlemen sometimes. Sadly, there do not seem to be many male carers compared to females. This could be due to them feeling overwhelmed and outnumbered by the ladies.

I have to say that I am not often shocked by what family members ask me. Some time ago, however, I was showing a family around; carers at this home had to answer phones and do admin work and organise home viewings at evenings and weekends because the company would not pay for reception staff for any more hours. This family said, 'How many of your staff members are foreign?' Now, yes, we did have a few foreign members of staff, but I feel managers need to be careful on this ground. Firstly, though, when I have been in the unfortunate situation of working with carers who are very poor at the job, they have probably more often been British than not. Many foreign nationals are lovely. The biggest problem is the language barrier, speaking and listening. When reading English, can they understand the drug names and dosages? Many of my patients cannot understand what I am saying, so working to understand another language could cause them frustration; how can this be dealt with?

One nurse upset a patient's relative once by saying to her she thought the family were all failures, because in that family's culture they have their loved ones live with them until their passing. We cannot let our own beliefs affect our judgement.

At the end of the day I do not think anyone will worry about who is looking after their loved one as long as they can see they are getting the care they need. I would rather have a whole home of foreign nationals that were good at their job than some of the English people who have let their residents and colleagues down.

Many people come fresh from college with their qualifications on paper but have never had the practical experience; one girl came to us to start and lasted half a day after realising she could not cope with bodily functions.

Staff warning: putting concerns down to dementia again

Too many carers I have worked with in the past have often said to me, 'The dementia is progressing; they've lost the plot.' The fact is that new or worsening confusion is quite often due to simple things. Delirium, confusion from dehydration, constipation and urine or chest infections can literally send people a bit daft. Sometimes this job is a bit like detective work. Tracking down the right solution will prevent unnecessary treatments.

Carers are the people who spend the most time with patients, so we are often the first ones to recognise changes in health to pass over to nursing staff. We need to remember that some patients are unable to tell us they have pains, so we need to spot them ourselves. Holding an area, agitated behaviour, rocking backwards and forwards, wincing when they move etc. can all be signs.

Families rely on us; now that their relative is in care, they should be confident that we will look after things. Sometimes, though, a relative may spot things that are unusual for their loved one. If this happens, we need to speak to a nurse about their findings; after all, they have known this person all their life. Remember we have been given the privilege of looking after the most precious people in the relatives' lives, so we have to be 100 per cent dedicated to their every need.

If confusion is indeed assessed to be progression of dementia, it is important to find ways both of helping our resident in any way we can and of supporting their family, who will also be told the news.

My hopes for this book

My hopes for this book are simple, really. I want people to realise the importance of good care in our society for our future patients. I want people in the care sector to think hard about whether they do their job right, or maybe people outside it to think about whether they can actually make this career choice.

I want all care companies and staff to stop and think about what is really needed for our patients and whether they are being given it.

Most importantly, I want people who are not listened to by managers to whistle-blow to the CQC so their patients' rights are upheld.

One definite thing is that people are living longer, our population is growing and there will always be a high number of people needing care. This guide is on what to look for, how to keep an eye on standards in a home and what to expect if your own loved one requires care.

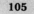

While many homes are not abusive physically, they are still providing inadequate care; if managers were actually truthful about what people's loved ones would receive for their money, many homes would not be filled. The care home is not a conveyer belt. A previous nursing manager told me once to feed them, wash them and toilet them; job done. 'Horrific' is the only way I can describe this attitude to the care of all those mums and dads in that home. We need to make sure that homes like this are exposed and have action taken, and that the good ones are praised. For goodness' sake, I spent more time bathing and grooming my dog than I was allowed to give each resident every day in previous homes.

I've witnessed poor care, abuse and good care in my years in a caring role. So many carers have said to me, 'I have witnessed this, I am not happy about that,' and have always been afraid to speak out. We have a duty of care to people's loved ones; managers have the ultimate responsibility of providing safe and good care for their residents. I have seen how hard it is, have experienced times when I have felt like I am banging my head against a brick wall. As you grow in experience it is frightening to realise how many situations you may have been in where care was very poor, or abuse was taking place.

Every manager should be open and honest. I have heard the 'my door is always open' claim in the past, but they forgot to add 'unless your concerns are about the residents' welfare, because I don't feel we need to act on those concerns'.

Many of our patients have no family, or the family that does come in see the whole dishonest front given by staff. We see, we know, we have the choice to act and not let someone suffer, yet so often in my past we were intimidated into not doing this; things were played down. To me, my patients are the most important thing about my job, and if I ever had a concern which was ignored there would be no silence; I would make my voice heard. I would do this if needed because all these people's families have trusted me to be their loved one's protector, and speaking up, we all know deep down, is sometimes the only way to get heard. I would rather upset staff than let someone suffer, because we are their only hope. So many care workers I have known have said to me they hope surveillance happens because they feel this is the only way managers will listen, and I find this very sad as well as frightening. One of my residents from eight years ago said to me, 'You are my guardian angel now as I have nobody else,' and this is why we cannot choose silence in response to bad care. Any family would thank you for being honest because many people do not know how to really see what goes on. We are relied on for everything.

I want to stamp out all poor care by presenting the view from someone on the front line. I never want my bad experiences to happen to anyone else. We can achieve this if we all just unite on a zero-tolerance approach to abuse, give praise and respect to all good staff and deal with issues quickly.

I want patients to be able to live not just exist.

Let's hear positive stories on how care homes are enriching people's lives, rather than seeing footage of abuse.

Let's make sure we include the family in their loved one's decisions and support them all the way through their loved one's care. Hopefully, if we achieve this, more and more relatives will be able to say to themselves and others, 'You know the care home so-and-so is in? That is a care home that really cares.'

I am always thinking of ways to improve quality of life

I have been in many care magazines for my Mediclipz invention for walking aids. Seeing the dementia problem and how it often restricted people from getting out in case they got lost, I came up with an idea for a device that I make myself, which is patent pending. Mediclipz are clips that contain a label with vital information about the patient, such as their name and contact details for their home, and can be attached to the tubing of walking aids and wheelchairs. Some care homes are using them to name mobility aids; this prevents people picking up the wrong aid and avoids having to use horrible sticky-taped paper names. You see so many dementia patients empty their pockets of house keys, money, ID etc. before they go out, but most take their walking aid. If the patient's details are clipped securely onto that walking aid, anyone who finds them lost will be able to help them get back to safety.

A voice for care workers and families of those in care

Through my experiences I have learned there are so many people who suffer in silence when they have concerns, often with nobody to talk to about their situations. I will be opening up a discussion forum on my book website (http://www.adzcreations.com) so like-minded people can share their experiences to do with care. Families of those in care, those who are carers themselves and other members of care home staff are all welcome to join. Basically anyone with experiences, positive or negative, and anyone who is passionate about turning care around to enhance the lives of people.

With thanks to the people who have supported me

With thanks to my loving husband and three beautiful children for supporting my beliefs and putting up with me behind pen and paper.

Every single staff member I work with works tire-lessly to do their best for every resident and their families. In my personal opinion, they have created the only place I have ever worked that I could trust with my loved ones if I needed to.

Lightning Source UK Ltd.
Milton Keynes UK
UKOW02f1805300814

237792UK00001B/20/P